CANCER DIET COOKBOOK FOR SENIORS

The complete guide with simple, quick and nourishing recipes to fight cancer and reclaim your health

Frank Douglas

This book is a heartfelt endeavor dedicated to providing support, nourishment, and comfort to those navigating the challenging journey of cancer in their golden years.

Cancer is a formidable opponent that affects people of all ages, but it can be particularly challenging for the elderly. As we age, our bodies become more vulnerable, and the physical and emotional toll of cancer can be intensified. In the face of such adversity, maintaining a balanced diet becomes paramount, as proper nutrition plays a vital role in supporting the body's ability to fight and heal.

In this book, we aim to empower cancer warriors and their caregivers with a collection of nourishing recipes specially crafted to meet the unique dietary needs of elderly individuals battling cancer. These recipes have been thoughtfully developed with a deep understanding of the challenges faced during this time. We have taken into account the common symptoms and side effects of cancer treatments, such as loss of appetite, taste changes, difficulty swallowing, and digestive issues, to create meals that are not only nutritious but also gentle on the body.

We understand that cooking can be overwhelming and time-consuming when faced with the demands of cancer care. Therefore, we have carefully selected recipes that are easy to prepare, using readily available ingredients. Whether you are a caregiver seeking to provide your loved one with nourishment or an elderly individual determined to maintain their strength, this book will serve as a valuable resource.

Throughout these pages, you will find a variety of dishes spanning from hearty soups and comforting stews to flavorful smoothies and easy-to-chew meals. Each recipe comes with clear instructions, accompanied by nutritional information to help you make informed choices about your dietary intake.

It is important to note that this book is not a substitute for medical advice or personalized dietary guidance. Every individual's journey with cancer is unique, and it is essential to consult with healthcare professionals for personalized nutritional recommendations.

We would like to express our deepest gratitude to the oncologists, dietitians, and caregivers who provided their expertise and insights, ensuring that the recipes included in this book align with the specific needs of elderly cancer warriors. Your unwavering dedication to the well-being of your patients and loved ones has been invaluable.

Above all, this book is a tribute to the strength, resilience, and unwavering spirit of cancer warriors. Your determination to fight, your bravery in the face of adversity, and your unwavering hope inspire us all. May these nourishing recipes bring you comfort, joy, and the sustenance needed for your journey.

Together, let us embark on this culinary voyage, offering sustenance and nourishment to those who need it most. Let us cook with love, compassion, and understanding, sharing meals that not only nourish the body but also warm the soul.

Chapter 1: Understanding Cancer and its impact on elderly individuals

Cancer is a complex disease that affects individuals of all ages, but its impact on the elderly population can be particularly challenging. As people age, their bodies become more susceptible to various health conditions, including cancer. In this article, we will delve into the subject of cancer in elderly individuals and explore the relevance of the book titled "Nourishing Recipes for Cancer Warriors: Cooking for Elderly Individuals" in providing valuable insights and guidance for managing cancer through nutrition.

Understanding Cancer in the Elderly:

Cancer is a disease characterized by the uncontrolled growth of abnormal cells in the body. It can occur in various forms and can affect different organs and tissues. With advancing age, the risk of developing cancer increases due to a combination of factors, including accumulated DNA damage, reduced immune function, and changes in hormone levels. Common types of cancer in the elderly include lung, breast, prostate, colorectal, and pancreatic cancer.

Cancer diagnosis and treatment can have a profound impact on the physical, emotional, and social well-being of elderly individuals. The aging body may respond differently to cancer treatments, making it more challenging to tolerate therapies such as chemotherapy or radiation. Additionally, coexisting health conditions and medications may complicate cancer management. Elderly cancer patients often experience fatigue, loss of appetite, weight loss, and increased vulnerability to infections.

Overview of cancer and its types

There are several types of cancer, each originating from different types of cells in the body. Here are some common types:

1. Breast Cancer: This type of cancer originates in the breast tissue, typically in the milk ducts or lobules. It affects both women and men, but it is more prevalent in women.

2. Lung Cancer: Lung cancer develops in the lung tissues, usually in the cells lining the air passages. It is strongly associated with smoking but can also occur in non-smokers.

3. Colorectal Cancer: Colorectal cancer affects the colon or rectum. It usually begins as small, noncancerous growths called polyps, which can become cancerous over time.

4. Prostate Cancer: Prostate cancer occurs in the prostate gland in men. It is one of the most common types of cancer in males and often grows slowly.

5. Pancreatic Cancer: Pancreatic cancer develops in the tissues of the pancreas, an organ responsible for producing digestive juices and hormones. It is known for its aggressive nature and tendency to be diagnosed at advanced stages.

6. Skin Cancer: Skin cancer affects the skin cells and is primarily caused by exposure to ultraviolet (UV) radiation from the sun or tanning beds. The most common types of skin cancer are basal cell carcinoma, squamous cell carcinoma, and melanoma.

7. Leukemia: Leukemia is a cancer of the blood cells, specifically the bone marrow and the lymphatic system. It is characterized by the overproduction of abnormal white blood cells, which affects the body's ability to fight infection.

8. Lymphoma: Lymphoma is a cancer that originates in the lymphatic system, which is responsible for fighting infections. There are two main types: Hodgkin lymphoma and non-Hodgkin lymphoma.

9. Ovarian Cancer: Ovarian cancer affects the ovaries, the reproductive organs in women. It often goes undetected until it has spread to the pelvis and abdomen, making it difficult to treat.

These are just a few examples of the many types of cancer that exist. Each type has its unique characteristics, treatment options, and challenges.

Challenges faced by elderly individuals with cancer

One of the primary challenges faced by elderly individuals with cancer is the impact of cancer treatments on their appetite and ability to eat. Chemotherapy, radiation therapy, and other cancer treatments can lead to a loss of appetite, taste changes, nausea, and difficulty swallowing. These issues make it challenging for elderly individuals to consume a well-balanced diet and maintain proper nutrition, which is crucial for their overall well-being and recovery. The book addresses these challenges by offering recipes that are easy to chew, digest, and packed with nutrients to support the body's healing process.

Another challenge for elderly individuals with cancer is the management of co-existing health conditions. Aging is often accompanied by chronic diseases such as diabetes, hypertension, or heart disease. These conditions can complicate cancer treatment and require careful management through dietary modifications. The book takes into account the specific dietary needs of individuals with multiple health conditions, providing recipes that are not only cancer-fighting but also considerate of other health concerns.

Mobility and physical limitations can also pose challenges for elderly individuals with cancer. Fatigue, weakness, and reduced mobility due to age or cancer treatments may affect their ability to shop for groceries, prepare meals, or even stand for long periods in the kitchen. The book addresses this challenge by offering practical tips and techniques for meal planning, prepping, and cooking that can make the process more manageable. It emphasizes the importance of simple and accessible ingredients, as well as strategies for batch cooking and freezing meals for convenience.

Social support and emotional well-being are also essential aspects of the cancer journey, especially for elderly individuals. Many older individuals face increased isolation and loneliness, which can be further exacerbated by a cancer diagnosis. The book recognizes the importance of food as a means of connection and support, providing not only recipes but also suggestions for creating a warm and nurturing environment during mealtime. It encourages the involvement of family members and caregivers in the cooking process, fostering a sense of togetherness and love through food.

Importance of nutrition in cancer treatment and recovery

Proper nutrition plays a critical role in supporting the overall health and well-being of individuals undergoing cancer treatment. Here are some key points to consider:

1. Maintaining strength and energy: Cancer treatments such as chemotherapy and radiation can often cause side effects like fatigue, nausea, and loss of appetite. Consuming a well-balanced diet that includes adequate calories, proteins, and healthy fats can help combat these side effects, improve energy levels, and maintain muscle mass.

2. Supporting immune function: Cancer treatment can weaken the immune system, making the body more susceptible to infections. A nutrient-rich diet that includes a variety of fruits, vegetables, whole grains, and lean proteins can provide essential vitamins, minerals, and antioxidants that support immune function and help fight off infections.

3. Managing treatment side effects: Certain nutrients and dietary strategies can help manage specific treatment-related side effects. For example, consuming ginger may alleviate nausea, while foods rich in fiber can help prevent or relieve constipation often associated with certain medications. The book may provide specific recipes and guidelines tailored to address these side effects.

4. Promoting healing and recovery: Cancer treatments can cause damage to healthy cells and tissues. Adequate nutrition, particularly with a focus on nutrient-dense foods, can help support the body's healing process and aid in tissue repair.

5. Enhancing overall well-being: Eating well during cancer treatment can have a positive impact on an individual's overall well-being. Good nutrition can help improve mood, reduce stress,

and promote a sense of control and empowerment during a challenging time.

Chapter 2: Nutritional guide for Cancer warriors

When it comes to fighting cancer, nutrition plays a crucial role in maintaining overall health, supporting the immune system, managing side effects of treatment, and promoting recovery. The recipes in this book are thoughtfully crafted to incorporate a wide range of nutrients, vitamins, minerals, and antioxidants that can aid in boosting the body's defenses and supporting the healing process.

Here are some key elements of the nutritional guide:

1. Balanced Macronutrients: The book emphasizes the importance of consuming a well-balanced diet that includes all three macronutrients—carbohydrates, proteins, and fats. These macronutrients provide the necessary energy and building blocks for the body to function optimally.

2. Whole Foods: The recipes in the book predominantly feature whole foods such as fruits, vegetables, whole grains, legumes, lean proteins, and healthy fats. These foods are rich in essential nutrients and phytochemicals, which have been shown to have anticancer properties.

3. Anti-Inflammatory Foods: Chronic inflammation is linked to the development and

progression of cancer. The nutritional guide suggests incorporating foods that have anti-inflammatory properties, such as turmeric, ginger, garlic, green leafy vegetables, berries, and nuts.

4. Antioxidant-Rich Ingredients: Antioxidants help protect the body's cells from damage caused by free radicals, which can contribute to the development of cancer. The book emphasizes including ingredients like colorful fruits and vegetables, herbs, spices, and certain nuts and seeds that are known for their high antioxidant content.

5. Adequate Hydration: Staying hydrated is vital for cancer patients, as it supports various bodily functions and helps alleviate certain treatment side effects. The guide recommends drinking plenty of fluids, including water, herbal teas, and broths, to maintain proper hydration.

6. Managing Side Effects: Cancer treatments often come with side effects that can affect appetite, taste, and digestion. The book offers suggestions and recipes specifically designed to address these issues, such as incorporating mild flavors, softer textures, and smaller, more frequent meals.

7. Personalization: Each individual's nutritional needs may vary based on their specific type of cancer, treatment plan, and overall health status. The nutritional guide encourages cancer warriors to work with their healthcare team or a registered dietitian to tailor the recipes and recommendations to their unique circumstances.

"Nourishing Recipes for Cancer Warriors" aims to provide cancer patients and their caregivers with a comprehensive nutritional resource that supports their overall well-being during their battle against cancer. By incorporating these nourishing recipes into their diet, cancer warriors can strive to optimize their nutrition and support their body's fight against the disease.

When it comes to cooking for elderly individuals with cancer, it is important to prioritize their nutritional needs and provide them with a well-rounded, nourishing diet. Here are some kitchen essentials that can help you create meals that are not only delicious but also supportive of their health:

1. Fresh Produce: Stock your kitchen with a variety of fresh fruits and vegetables. Opt for vibrant colors, as they indicate high levels of essential vitamins, minerals, and antioxidants. Include leafy greens, cruciferous vegetables like broccoli and cauliflower, berries, citrus fruits, and other seasonal produce.

2. Whole Grains: Choose whole grain options like brown rice, quinoa, oats, and whole wheat bread. These provide important dietary fiber, which aids digestion and helps maintain a healthy weight.

3. Lean Proteins: Incorporate lean sources of protein such as skinless poultry, fish, legumes, tofu, and low-fat dairy products. Protein is crucial for tissue repair and immune function.

4. Healthy Fats: Include healthy fats like avocados, nuts, seeds, and olive oil. These provide essential fatty acids and help absorb fat-soluble vitamins.

5. Herbs and Spices: Enhance the flavor of dishes using herbs and spices. They not only add taste but also offer potential health benefits. Turmeric, ginger, garlic, cinnamon, and basil are known for their anti-inflammatory and antioxidant properties.

6. Low-Sodium Broths and Stocks: Using low-sodium options as the base for soups and stews can add flavor without excessive salt, which is important for individuals with cancer who may have specific dietary restrictions.

7. Blender or Food Processor: These appliances are useful for making smoothies, purees, and soups with a smoother consistency, especially for individuals with difficulty chewing or swallowing.

8. Non-Stick Cookware: Opt for non-stick cookware to minimize the need for excess oil or fat during cooking, making meals healthier overall.

9. Nutritional Supplements: Consult with healthcare professionals about the possibility of including specific nutritional supplements that may be beneficial for the individual's condition.

10. Portion Control Tools: Measuring cups, spoons, and a food scale can help ensure that portion sizes are appropriate and that the individual receives the right amount of nutrients.

11. Safe Food Handling Tools: Maintain good hygiene and food safety practices by having separate cutting boards, knives, and utensils for raw and cooked foods. This helps minimize the risk of foodborne illnesses.

Remember, it is essential to consult with healthcare professionals or a registered dietitian who can provide personalized dietary recommendations based on the specific needs and conditions of the elderly individual with cancer.

In the journey of battling cancer, maintaining a nourishing and balanced diet is essential for overall well-being. Breakfast, being the most important meal of the day, provides the necessary energy to kickstart the morning and support the body's healing process. This chapter presents a selection of quick and easy breakfast recipes specially designed for cancer warriors.These recipes focus on providing essential nutrients, incorporating cancer-fighting ingredients, and being easy to prepare, ensuring a nutritious and delicious start to the day.

Berry Blast Smoothie:

Ingredients:

1 cup mixed berries (strawberries, blueberries, raspberries)

1 ripe banana

1 cup almond milk (or any other non-dairy milk)

1 tablespoon chia seeds

1 tablespoon honey (optional)

Instructions:

Blend all the ingredients together until smooth.

Pour into a glass and enjoy the refreshing and antioxidant-rich Berry Blast Smoothie, packed with vitamins and minerals to boost your immune system.

Ingredients:

1 ripe avocado

2 slices of whole-grain bread

1 teaspoon turmeric powder

Pinch of salt and pepper

Fresh lemon juice

Instructions:

Mash the avocado in a bowl and add a squeeze of fresh lemon juice.

Toast the slices of bread until golden brown.

Spread the mashed avocado on the toasted bread.

Sprinkle turmeric powder, salt, and pepper on top.

Serve this vibrant and anti-inflammatory Avocado Toast with Turmeric, providing healthy fats, fiber, and powerful antioxidants.

Ingredients:

1 cup cooked quinoa

1/2 cup Greek yogurt (or dairy-free alternative)

1 tablespoon honey

1/4 cup mixed nuts and seeds (such as almonds, walnuts, pumpkin seeds, chia seeds)

Fresh fruits (e.g., sliced banana, berries, or diced mango)

Cinnamon (optional)

Instructions:

In a bowl, combine cooked quinoa, Greek yogurt, and honey.

Top it with mixed nuts and seeds, fresh fruits, and a sprinkle of cinnamon.

This Quinoa Breakfast Bowl is not only packed with protein but also provides a variety of essential nutrients, including fiber, vitamins, and minerals.

Ingredients:

4 eggs

1/4 cup chopped vegetables (e.g., spinach, bell peppers, onions, mushrooms)

Salt and pepper to taste

Grated cheese (optional)

Instructions:

Preheat the oven to 350°F (175°C) and grease a muffin tin.

In a bowl, whisk the eggs and season with salt and pepper.

Add the chopped vegetables and mix well.

Pour the mixture into the greased muffin tin, filling each cup about 3/4 full.

If desired, sprinkle grated cheese on top.

Bake for 15-20 minutes until the egg muffins are set and slightly golden.

Enjoy these Veggie Egg Muffins, which provide protein, vitamins, and minerals while allowing for a quick grab-and-go breakfast option.

In conclusion, Starting the day with a nourishing breakfast is vital for cancer warriors. These quick and easy recipes are aimed to provide essential nutrients, incorporate cancer-fighting ingredients, and be simple to prepare. By enjoying these breakfast options, cancer warriors can fuel their bodies, support their immune systems, and enjoy delicious and satisfying meals to begin their day with positivity and strength.

Chapter 5: Nourishing soups and Healing broths

Nourishing soups and healing broths play a vital role in the lives of individuals battling cancer, often referred to as "cancer warriors." These recipes are specifically designed to provide nourishment, support the immune system, and aid in the healing process. The importance of proper nutrition cannot be overstated during this challenging time, as it helps maintain strength, manage side effects of treatments, and promote overall well-being.

When it comes to creating nourishing recipes for cancer warriors, soups and broths offer a multitude of benefits. They are easy to digest, gentle on the stomach, and can be customized to meet specific dietary needs and taste preferences. Moreover, they provide a concentrated source of essential nutrients, vitamins, and minerals that support the body's healing process.

Key elements to consider when preparing nourishing soups and healing broths for cancer warriors:

Nutrient-Dense Ingredients: Incorporate a variety of fresh, whole foods into the recipes. Include nutrient-rich vegetables such as leafy greens, cruciferous vegetables (broccoli, cauliflower, Brussels sprouts), root vegetables (carrots, sweet potatoes), and medicinal mushrooms like shiitake or maitake. These ingredients provide vitamins, minerals, and antioxidants that support the immune system and help combat fatigue.

Homemade Broths: Start with a homemade broth as the base of your soups. Bone broth, vegetable broth, or mushroom broth can be prepared by simmering bones or vegetables for an extended period, extracting valuable nutrients and minerals. These broths are not only rich in flavor but also provide easily absorbable nutrients, including collagen, amino acids, and minerals that support gut health and aid in the healing process.

Protein-Rich Additions: Protein is crucial for cell repair and regeneration. Enhance the nutritional content of your soups and broths by adding lean protein sources such as cooked chicken, turkey, fish, or plant-based options like beans, lentils, or tofu. These additions offer essential amino acids and help maintain muscle mass during cancer treatment.

Anti-Inflammatory Herbs and Spices: Incorporate herbs and spices known for their anti-inflammatory properties, such as turmeric, ginger, garlic, and fresh herbs like cilantro or parsley. These ingredients not only add depth of flavor but also provide potential health benefits, including reducing inflammation and aiding digestion.

Easy-to-Digest Texture: Ensure the soups and broths have a smooth and easily digestible texture. This can be achieved by blending the ingredients or using a strainer to remove any fibrous components. Adjust the thickness and consistency based on individual preferences and dietary restrictions.

Hydration and Sipping Broths: Cancer treatments can sometimes cause dehydration and a loss of appetite. Create sipping broths by simmering vegetables, herbs, and spices in water to create a flavorful, nutrient-rich drink that can be sipped throughout the day. These broths can help maintain hydration and provide essential nutrients even when the appetite is diminished.

It's important to note that while nourishing soups and healing broths can complement cancer treatments, they should not replace medical advice or treatments prescribed by healthcare professionals. Always consult with a healthcare provider or a registered dietitian before making significant changes to the diet, especially during cancer treatment.

Nourishing soups and healing broths offer a comforting and nutrient-packed option for cancer warriors. These recipes can be tailored to individual needs, providing essential nutrients, supporting the immune system, and aiding in the healing process. By incorporating nutrient-dense ingredients, homemade broths, lean proteins, anti-inflammatory herbs and spices, and focusing on easy-to-digest textures, these recipes can contribute to overall well-being and nourishment during the cancer journey.

Chapter 6: Nurturing main course dishes

When it comes to battling cancer, proper nutrition plays a crucial role in supporting the overall well-being and strength of cancer warriors. A well-balanced diet can help manage treatment side effects, boost the immune system, and promote healing. Main course dishes, in particular, provide an excellent opportunity to create nourishing recipes that are both delicious and supportive of the body's needs during cancer treatment.

Focus on Whole Foods: Incorporate a variety of whole foods into main course dishes to ensure a broad spectrum of nutrients. Opt for lean proteins such as fish, poultry, tofu, and legumes, which provide essential amino acids and help maintain muscle mass. Including a generous serving of colorful vegetables in each dish adds vital vitamins, minerals, and antioxidants.

Prioritize Plant-Based Ingredients: Plant-based meals have gained recognition for their potential health benefits, including their role in cancer prevention and management. Utilize a wide range of plant-based ingredients like leafy greens, cruciferous vegetables, whole grains, and nuts to create nourishing main courses. These ingredients are rich in fiber, vitamins, minerals, and phytochemicals, which contribute to overall well-being.

Emphasize Anti-Inflammatory Ingredients: Chronic inflammation can be a contributing factor in cancer development and progression. By incorporating anti-inflammatory foods into main course dishes, cancer warriors can help reduce inflammation and support their immune system. Turmeric, ginger, garlic, onions, and green leafy vegetables are excellent choices to include in recipes due to their anti-inflammatory properties.

Choose Healthy Cooking Techniques: Opt for cooking techniques that retain the maximum nutritional value of the ingredients while enhancing flavor. Steaming, baking, grilling, and sautéing with minimal oil are great options. These methods help preserve the natural goodness of the ingredients without adding unnecessary fats or calories.

Integrate Cancer-Fighting Herbs and Spices: Many herbs and spices have potent cancer-fighting properties and can enhance the taste of main course dishes. Incorporate herbs like rosemary, thyme, oregano, and basil, which are rich in antioxidants and possess anti-cancer properties.

Spices such as turmeric, cinnamon, cumin, and ginger offer both flavor and potential health benefits.

Customize to Individual Needs: Cancer treatments can vary, and individual dietary requirements may change over time. It is crucial to work closely with healthcare professionals, such as oncologists and registered dietitians, to tailor recipes and main course dishes to meet specific nutritional needs. This customization ensures that the dishes are suitable for the person's treatment plan, any potential side effects, and their overall health goals.

Prioritize Hydration: Adequate hydration is essential for cancer warriors to support their overall well-being and manage treatment-related side effects. Incorporate hydrating ingredients into main course dishes, such as soups, stews, and casseroles that include broth or other liquid bases. Additionally, encourage the consumption of water and other hydrating beverages throughout the day.

Remember, each cancer journey is unique, and it's essential to consult with healthcare professionals and registered dietitians to develop a personalized nutrition plan. Nurturing main course dishes can be an opportunity to create nourishing recipes that not only provide essential nutrients but also satisfy the taste buds and support the overall well-being of cancer warriors.

Chapter 7: Sides and Salads for optimal nutrition

When it comes to nourishing recipes for cancer warriors, incorporating sides and salads can play a vital role in providing optimal nutrition and supporting overall well-being. These dishes can contribute a wide range of nutrients, antioxidants, and phytochemicals that promote immune function, aid in recovery, and support the body during cancer treatment. Let's explore some ideas for sides and salads that can be beneficial for cancer warriors.

Roasted Vegetable Medley:

Roasting a variety of colorful vegetables like broccoli, carrots, bell peppers, and Brussels sprouts not only enhances their natural flavors but also preserves their nutritional value. Roasted vegetables are rich in fiber, vitamins, minerals, and antioxidants that can help reduce inflammation and strengthen the immune system.

Quinoa Salad:

Quinoa is a nutrient-dense grain that is high in protein and fiber. Combine cooked quinoa with an assortment of fresh vegetables such as cucumbers, cherry tomatoes, spinach, and herbs like parsley or cilantro. Add a light dressing made from lemon juice, olive oil, and herbs for a refreshing and satisfying salad. Quinoa provides essential amino acids, while vegetables contribute vitamins, minerals, and antioxidants.

Kale and Avocado Salad:

Kale is a powerhouse of nutrients, including vitamins A, C, and K, as well as minerals like calcium and iron. Combine finely chopped kale with ripe avocado slices, cherry tomatoes, red onion, and a sprinkle of nuts or seeds. Toss with a lemon or balsamic vinaigrette to create a nutritious and flavorful salad rich in antioxidants and healthy fats.

Lentil Soup:

A warm and comforting lentil soup can be a nutritious side dish for cancer warriors. Lentils are packed with plant-based protein, fiber, and essential minerals. Combine lentils with a variety of vegetables such as carrots, celery, and onions, along with flavorful herbs and spices like turmeric and cumin. This hearty soup provides a good balance of protein, fiber, and micronutrients.

Rainbow Fruit Salad:

Fruits are excellent sources of vitamins, minerals, and antioxidants. Create a vibrant fruit salad by combining a colorful array of fruits like berries, citrus fruits, kiwi, and melons. This salad not only satisfies the taste buds but also provides essential nutrients and hydration.

Remember to consider individual dietary restrictions and sensitivities when preparing these dishes. Additionally, it is advisable to consult a registered dietitian or healthcare professional for personalized nutrition guidance tailored to the specific needs of cancer warriors.

When it comes to battling cancer, maintaining proper nutrition and energy levels is crucial. Cancer treatments can often cause side effects like fatigue, nausea, and loss of appetite, making it challenging to meet nutritional needs. That's why incorporating nourishing snacks and small bites into the diet of cancer warriors becomes essential. These snacks provide sustained energy, vital nutrients, and help combat the side effects of cancer treatments.

Here are some nourishing snack ideas for cancer warriors to boost their energy levels and support their overall well-being:

Nut Butter and Banana Wrap:

Spread a tablespoon of your favorite nut butter (such as almond butter or peanut butter) on a whole wheat or gluten-free wrap. Place a sliced banana on top and roll it up. This snack offers a combination of healthy fats, protein, and carbohydrates, providing sustained energy and essential nutrients.

Protein-Packed Energy Balls:

Prepare energy balls using a combination of nuts (such as almonds, walnuts, or cashews), dates, and a protein-rich ingredient like chia seeds, hemp hearts, or protein powder. These bite-sized snacks are easy to make, portable, and packed with nutrients, including fiber, healthy fats, and antioxidants.

Greek Yogurt Parfait:

Layer Greek yogurt with fresh berries, a sprinkle of granola or nuts, and a drizzle of honey or maple syrup. Greek yogurt is an excellent source of protein, while berries provide antioxidants and fiber. This snack is not only delicious but also supports digestion and provides a sustained energy boost.

Avocado Toast:

Spread mashed avocado on whole grain bread and top it with a sprinkle of sea salt, black pepper, and other toppings of your choice. Avocado is a nutrient-dense fruit that provides healthy fats, vitamins, and minerals. This snack is quick to prepare and offers a satisfying combination of flavors and textures.

Veggie Sticks with Hummus:

Slice a variety of fresh vegetables such as carrots, cucumbers, bell peppers, and celery into sticks. Pair them with a flavorful hummus dip. This snack is rich in fiber, vitamins, and minerals, and the combination of vegetables and hummus provides a balance of carbohydrates, protein, and healthy fats.

Quinoa Salad Cups:

Prepare a quinoa salad by combining cooked quinoa with diced vegetables, herbs, and a light vinaigrette dressing. Spoon the salad into small lettuce cups or use mini muffin tins to create bite-sized portions. Quinoa is a protein-rich grain that offers sustained energy, while the vegetables provide essential nutrients and antioxidants.

Smoothies:

Blend together a combination of fruits, leafy greens, yogurt or milk, and a spoonful of nut butter or seeds. Smoothies are an excellent way to incorporate a variety of nutrient-dense ingredients into a single snack. They are easy to digest, hydrating, and provide a quick energy boost.

Remember, it's crucial to consult with a healthcare professional or a registered dietitian who specializes in oncology nutrition to tailor these snack ideas to your specific needs and preferences. They can provide personalized recommendations and ensure the snacks align with your treatment plan and overall dietary requirements.

By incorporating nourishing snacks and small bites like these into your diet, you can support your energy levels, enhance overall nutrition, and promote well-being as you navigate your cancer journey.

Chapter 9: Comfort desserts for a sweet treat

Sweet treats can play a significant role in providing comfort and a sense of pleasure during challenging times. Comfort desserts, specifically designed to be nourishing and supportive, can uplift the spirits and provide a delightful respite for those undergoing cancer treatment. Here are a few ideas for comforting desserts that are both delicious and nourishing.

Berry Parfait:

A berry parfait combines the goodness of fresh berries with layers of creamy yogurt or coconut milk and a sprinkle of crunchy granola. Berries are rich in antioxidants, vitamins, and fiber, which can support overall health. The creaminess of yogurt or coconut milk adds a luscious texture to the dessert, while the granola provides a satisfying crunch.

Avocado Chocolate Mousse:

Avocado chocolate mousse is a decadent and velvety dessert that can bring joy to anyone's palate. Avocados are packed with healthy fats, fiber, and essential nutrients. Blending ripe avocados with dark cocoa powder, a touch of sweetener like maple syrup or honey, and a hint of vanilla creates a smooth and indulgent mousse. This dessert offers a dose of healthy fats and antioxidants, while satisfying chocolate cravings.

Chia Seed Pudding:

Chia seed pudding is a versatile dessert that can be customized to suit individual tastes. Chia seeds are an excellent source of omega-3 fatty acids, fiber, and protein. By combining chia seeds with a liquid such as almond milk, coconut milk, or dairy milk, and adding flavors like vanilla, cinnamon, or cocoa powder, you can create a creamy pudding. Allow the mixture to sit overnight to achieve a pudding-like consistency. Top it with fresh fruit or a sprinkle of nuts for added flavor and texture.

Baked Apples with Cinnamon:

Baked apples with cinnamon offer a warm and comforting dessert option. Apples are rich in fiber, vitamins, and antioxidants. Simply core the apples and fill them with a mixture of cinnamon, honey or maple syrup, and a small amount of butter or coconut oil. Bake until tender and fragrant. The result is a soft, sweet, and aromatic dessert that pairs beautifully with a dollop of Greek yogurt or a sprinkle of chopped nuts.

Banana nice cream is a healthy alternative to traditional ice cream. Peel and freeze ripe bananas, then blend them until smooth and creamy. The natural sweetness of bananas creates a delectable base, and you can add other ingredients like frozen berries, cocoa powder, or a spoonful of nut butter for additional flavor variations. The result is a creamy and refreshing dessert that is naturally sweet and full of potassium and fiber.

Remember, these comfort desserts are intended to be nourishing and supportive while still offering a delightful treat. They can be enjoyed by cancer warriors as part of a well-balanced diet, providing not only a moment of indulgence but also valuable nutrients to support their overall well-being.

Chapter 10: Special Dietary considerations

Special dietary considerations play a crucial role in supporting the nutritional needs and overall well-being of cancer warriors. While undergoing cancer treatment, individuals may experience various side effects such as loss of appetite, taste changes, nausea, vomiting, and difficulty swallowing. These challenges can make it difficult for cancer patients to maintain a healthy diet and meet their nutritional requirements. Therefore, creating nourishing recipes specifically designed for cancer warriors requires careful consideration of their dietary needs and preferences.

Important dietary considerations to keep in mind when developing nourishing recipes for cancer warriors:

Adequate calorie and nutrient intake: Cancer treatment can increase the body's energy and nutrient requirements. It is important to include nutrient-dense ingredients to ensure that patients receive sufficient calories, proteins, healthy fats, vitamins, and minerals. Lean proteins, whole grains, fruits, vegetables, and healthy fats like avocados and nuts can provide essential nutrients while being gentle on the digestive system.

Hydration: Staying hydrated is crucial for cancer patients, especially if they are experiencing vomiting or diarrhea due to treatment. Including hydrating ingredients such as soups, broths, smoothies, and herbal teas can help maintain fluid balance and prevent dehydration.

Soft and easy-to-digest foods: Many cancer patients may experience difficulty swallowing or have sensitive oral tissues due to treatment. Opting for soft, pureed, or blended foods can make it easier to consume essential nutrients. Soups, smoothies, pureed vegetables, and well-cooked grains are examples of foods that are gentle on the digestive system.

Balanced fiber intake: A balanced fiber intake is important for maintaining healthy digestion. However, some cancer treatments may cause digestive issues, such as diarrhea or constipation. Including soluble fibers found in fruits, vegetables, and whole grains can help regulate bowel movements and promote healthy digestion.

Managing taste changes: Cancer treatments can alter taste buds and lead to changes in taste perception, making certain foods unappealing or causing a metallic taste in the mouth.

Experimenting with different flavors, spices, and textures can help enhance the taste of dishes and make them more enjoyable. For example, using herbs, citrus juices, and mild spices can add flavor to meals without overwhelming the palate.

Anti-inflammatory foods: Chronic inflammation can be present in cancer patients, and consuming anti-inflammatory foods may help reduce inflammation and support overall health. Foods rich in omega-3 fatty acids (such as fatty fish and walnuts), colorful fruits and vegetables, turmeric, ginger, and green tea are known for their anti-inflammatory properties.

Individual preferences and dietary restrictions: It's essential to consider individual preferences, food aversions, and dietary restrictions when creating nourishing recipes for cancer warriors. Collaborating with healthcare professionals and dietitians can help develop personalized meal plans that address specific dietary needs and optimize the patient's nutritional intake.

Remember that each cancer patient's needs and preferences may vary, so it's important to tailor recipes to individual requirements. Consulting with healthcare professionals and registered dietitians who specialize in oncology nutrition can provide valuable guidance and ensure that the recipes meet the specific dietary considerations of cancer warriors.

Emotional and psychological support is a crucial aspect of holistic care for individuals fighting cancer. Alongside medical treatments and nourishing recipes, providing support to cancer warriors can greatly enhance their overall well-being and contribute to their healing journey. Nourishing recipes, specifically tailored to their nutritional needs, can serve as a powerful tool to boost physical strength and maintain a positive mindset. Let's explore how emotional and psychological support can be integrated with nourishing recipes to empower cancer warriors.

Creating a Supportive Environment: The process of battling cancer can be emotionally challenging, and cancer warriors need a supportive environment where they feel safe to express their thoughts and emotions. Loved ones, friends, and support groups can play a vital role in creating this environment by offering a listening ear, providing encouragement, and offering practical help. Encouraging cancer warriors to share their experiences, fears, and triumphs can help alleviate emotional burdens and foster a sense of belonging.

Promoting Mindfulness and Stress Reduction: Stress and anxiety are common experiences for cancer warriors, and managing these emotions is crucial for their well-being. Incorporating mindfulness techniques, such as deep breathing exercises, meditation, and gentle yoga, can help reduce stress levels. Encourage cancer warriors to engage in these practices alongside preparing nourishing recipes. Mindful cooking and savoring meals can help create a sense of calm and enhance the overall culinary experience.

Empowering with Nutritional Education: Educating cancer warriors about the importance of nutrition and its impact on their health is empowering. Providing them with information about the benefits of specific ingredients and how they can support their bodies during treatment can help them make informed choices. Offering guidance on ingredient substitutions, portion sizes, and meal planning can enhance their confidence in preparing nourishing recipes and maintaining a balanced diet.

Encouraging Creative Expression: Creative outlets, such as writing, painting, or crafting, can be therapeutic for cancer warriors. Encourage them to explore their creativity and express their emotions through these mediums. Alongside the creative process, incorporating nourishing ingredients into their recipes can serve as a sensory experience, providing comfort and satisfaction.

Celebrating Milestones and Achievements: Marking milestones and celebrating achievements, no matter how small, is vital in the cancer journey. Commemorate moments of strength, progress, and resilience by preparing special nourishing recipes. These celebratory meals can serve as a reminder of their journey and offer an opportunity for cancer warriors to reflect on their accomplishments and garner support from loved ones.

Connecting with Support Groups: Engaging with support groups, both in-person and online, can provide cancer warriors with a sense of community and understanding. These groups offer a platform to share experiences, exchange nourishing recipes, and provide emotional support. Encourage cancer warriors to participate actively in these communities, as they can find solace in the shared experiences of others and build valuable connections.

Emotional and psychological support is a crucial component of the care provided to cancer warriors. Integrating this support with nourishing recipes can create a holistic approach that addresses both the physical and emotional needs of individuals fighting cancer. By creating a supportive environment, promoting mindfulness, empowering through nutritional education, encouraging creative expression, celebrating milestones, and connecting with support groups, we can nurture the well-being of cancer warriors, helping them navigate their journey with strength and resilience.

Chapter 12: Conclusion

In the face of a cancer diagnosis, individuals become warriors in a battle against an often overwhelming enemy. Alongside medical treatments and therapies, nutrition plays a vital role in supporting their overall health and well-being. Nourishing recipes specifically designed for cancer warriors have emerged as a powerful tool, empowering individuals to take charge of their diet and optimize their journey towards healing.

Throughout this exploration of nourishing recipes for cancer warriors, we have witnessed the profound impact that food choices can have on a person's physical and emotional well-being. From reducing treatment side effects to enhancing the body's ability to fight cancer cells, nutrition has emerged as a cornerstone of comprehensive cancer care.

One of the key aspects of nourishing recipes for cancer warriors is their focus on providing essential nutrients while considering the specific dietary needs and challenges faced by individuals undergoing cancer treatment. These recipes emphasize the consumption of whole, unprocessed foods, rich in vitamins, minerals, antioxidants, and phytochemicals. By incorporating ingredients such as fruits, vegetables, whole grains, lean proteins, and healthy fats, these recipes promote overall health and support the body's healing processes.

Moreover, nourishing recipes for cancer warriors go beyond mere sustenance; they aim to create meals that are not only nutritious but also flavorful, satisfying, and enjoyable. The culinary aspect of these recipes plays a crucial role in promoting appetite and combating the loss of taste or appetite often associated with cancer treatments. By offering a diverse range of flavors and textures, these recipes help cancer warriors maintain a positive relationship with food and find pleasure in eating, even during challenging times.

Furthermore, the availability of nourishing recipes for cancer warriors has been greatly enhanced by the accessibility of information and resources through various platforms. Online communities, cookbooks, and support groups have become invaluable sources of guidance and inspiration, connecting individuals on their cancer journey and fostering a sense of community. The sharing of personal stories, experiences, and recipes has created a supportive environment that empowers cancer warriors to experiment, adapt, and customize their meals based on their unique preferences and needs.

It is essential to recognize that nourishing recipes for cancer warriors do not replace medical advice or treatments prescribed by healthcare professionals. Instead, they serve as a complementary tool, enabling individuals to actively participate in their own healing process. By making informed food choices and incorporating these recipes into their daily lives, cancer warriors gain a sense of control, confidence, and empowerment, knowing that they are actively contributing to their overall well-being.

Nourishing recipes for cancer warriors offer a holistic approach to support individuals throughout their cancer journey. By providing nutrient-dense meals that are both delicious and nourishing, these recipes empower individuals to take an active role in their health and well-being. The power of food, coupled with the support of a community, helps cancer warriors nourish their bodies, nurture their souls, and face their battle with strength and resilience.